HOW TO EAT RAW ON THE CHEAP

We tell ourselves a lot of excuses, especially when it comes to our eating habits. Maybe we had a difficult day and we say to ourselves, for example: "an extra ice cream why not? A chocolate maybe?" And our health and weight get worse.

We think that eating healthy and feeling good requires too much effort and sacrifice. I can assure you that this is absolutely not the case!

It is about re-educating our palate to the fresh and genuine flavors of fruit and vegetables; it's about learning how to prepare food again, and it's much easier than you might think!

Personally, it took me four days of total raw food to eliminate most of the cravings for cooked food I had, and even if I'm not 100% on raw food, I absolutely don't miss it.

The preparation of meals often takes me half the time of cooked food if not less!

So where is the problem? Why did I go back to eating cooked food for a year before throwing myself into raw food again?

Two reasons:

1) lack of variety in food, because I did not know enough recipes to allow me to vary my diet

2) because I believed that to be on a raw food diet took too much money and I was not in excellent financial position.

After almost a year in which my weight has increased and my breath and my energy have decreased, I have started looking for a way to return to raw food without spending more than 8 euros a day to eat, and often much less. .

The result is this book with which I want to share my experiences and discoveries with you.

HOW TO EAT RAW ON THE CHEAP

We tell ourselves a lot of excuses, especially when it comes to our eating habits. Maybe we had a difficult day and we say to ourselves, for example: "an extra ice cream why not? A chocolate maybe?" And our health and weight get worse.

We think that eating healthy and feeling good requires too much effort and sacrifice. I can assure you that this is absolutely not the case!

It is about re-educating our palate to the fresh and genuine flavors of fruit and vegetables; it's about learning how to prepare food again, and it's much easier than you might think!

Personally, it took me four days of total raw food to eliminate most of the cravings for cooked food I had, and even if I'm not 100% on raw food, I absolutely don't miss it.

The preparation of meals often takes me half the time of cooked food if not less!

So where is the problem? Why did I go back to eating cooked food for a year before throwing myself into raw food again?

Two reasons:

1) lack of variety in food, because I did not know enough recipes to allow me to vary my diet

2) because I believed that to be on a raw food diet took too much money and I was not in excellent financial position.

After almost a year in which my weight has increased and my breath and my energy have decreased, I have started looking for a way to return to raw food without spending more than 8 euros a day to eat, and often much less. .

The result is this book with which I want to share my experiences and discoveries with you.

F.A.Q.

Don't I have to buy a new kitchen?

Let's start with the kitchen: what do you need? I can tell you right away that if you want to eat raw food and spend little, you have to buy very few things. Even if you have been told that it takes expensive kitchen equipment to be "real" raw food, this is absolutely not the case. In reality, a fork, a knife and a plate would be enough but you would soon get bored with so little and you would go back to eating cooked food! So here are some tools that I consider essential:

1) Spiralizer. It is an essential tool for making spaghetti-like zucchini and carrots in no time. The one I use is from Gefu, but they can also be found at the flea markets. Average cost: from 10 to 22 euros 2) Blender. This will be used to prepare both smoothies and sauces and soups. While the blender you already own may be fine, as many of you already know, most blenders tend not to work smoothly and often break down prematurely. The best blenders are very expensive, like the famous Vitamix which goes for 600 euros, but I found an excellent balance between quality and price with the Dualetto blender, which costs from 22 to 40 euros including shipping. This blender, having the motor above two blades and two trays horizontally under the blender, is much better than traditional blenders and lasts much longer. Vitamix or similar can only serve you if you are a perfectionist or if you are a raw food chef!

3) Peeler. Essential for removing the peel from vegetables and fruit, especially when we don't buy organic. Average cost: from 1 to 5 euros.

4) Centrifuge or cotton or linen bag, new and undyed. Smoothies are excellent, but sometimes they are not suitable for certain preparations, such as almond milk, or sometimes a carrot centrifuge contains too much pulp for our taste! Furthermore, after some time following the raw food diet we may want to clean up further and to send our stomach on vacation and at the same time filling up with vitamins, minerals and enzymes. In this case we can adopt for a few days or even a month or two a diet of only fruit and vegetable centrifuges in quantities of even 3 or 4 liters per day,

eliminating fiber. Alternatively, you can also use a new, undyed cotton or linen bag to squeeze the pulp and separate it from the juice. Although this may be a feasible alternative if you occasionally use centrifuges or the like, it is not practical if you decide to make 3 liters of juice a day! Cost of centrifuge: from 30 to 100 euros depends on the type.

For those who also want to make wheatgrass juices though, the cost can also reach 300 euros

5) A good knife. If you have some extra money to spend you can get a ceramic knife that does not change the taste of food and does not oxidize vitamins like a steel knife, but it is not absolutely essential.

6) Coffee grinder. Very useful for finely chopping nuts and seeds before adding them to recipes. Not essential but it is worth buying it, since it costs about 20 euros.

7) Let's talk about an instrument, definitely not essential if you want to spend little, but which can make your diet much more varied: the dryer.

In practice this is similar to an oven, often ventilated, which in raw food is kept at a temperature not exceeding 40 degrees Celsius, so that enzymes are not destroyed and the vitamins contained in foods

are not denatured, (in recipes with ingredients that contain a lot of water such as biscuits and raw bread it is recommended instead to raise the temperature to 60 degrees until the water has evaporated completely and then to decrease it to 40 degrees, since during the evaporation of the water the food does not exceed 40 degrees.

This way also avoids the formation of mold and bacteria. The important thing is that the dryer is ventilated). Good dryers generally cost a lot and the only one I can recommend is the Excalibur.

Unfortunately, the cost is between 330 and 400 euros. If you feel like doing this shopping, I highly recommend the 9-shelf one, to use it to the fullest and to save on electricity by drying more things simultaneously (in fact you can put both sweet and savory things to dry on different shelves and the flavors generally do not mix). The dryer does not consume much electricity, less than an oven, but it needs to be kept on for much longer, sometimes from 6 to 12 or 24 hours!

Alternatively a very economical dryer to try is Dcg Eltronic Dryer Fd1065. The price is around 50 euros with shipping costs on ebay and other sites

There are two alternatives to the dryer: the simplest is not to use it as I do at the moment and concentrate, as in the vast majority of this book, on recipes that do not require it or that can be good even without its use.

The second option is to build one yourself, there are several sites with instructions for doing this. However, remember to choose a scheme with a fan and a front closure as otherwise the food may not dry out uniformly and form molds. Below are some sites in English and Italian for those who want to try their hand at DIY: http: //

courtneymeier.artifex.org/dehydrator/Electric_food_dehydrator_plans.pdf

http://www.squidoo.com/solar-food-dehydrator (solar dryer)
http://vegetarian.lovetoknow.com/Build_Your_Own_Food_Dehydrat

or

http://www.instructables.com/id/Inexpensive-Food-Dehydrator-with-Recycled-Parts/

What to buy to save money?

There are some pantry or fridge ingredients that I consider essential in the raw food diet, some for their nutritional value, others to vary the diet so as not to get bored, and others for both reasons. After a small initial expense to buy them you will find that they last a long time because often you don't need large quantities. They can be found easily in organic shops and supermarkets. Some of them can be found on raw food sites.

Nutritional yeast

It recalls the taste of cheese, and is very useful for preparing raw cheeses. Contains B vitamins and enzymes. Cost: from 4 to 5 euros for a 200 gr bag.

Tahini

It is obtained from sesame seeds. The best tasting in my opinion is the dark Tahini (even if it is not really raw because the seeds are toasted). It can be added to different dishes for a strong flavor. Rich in B vitamins, minerals such as iron, calcium, magnesium, phosphorus and zinc and essential fatty acids, in particular oleic and linoleic acids. Cost: from 4 to 7 euros for 250gr.

Spices

Essential for variety and for many preparations.

Agave syrup / Lucuma powder / Xylitol / Stevia Natural and raw sweeteners. We all know the dangers of sugar, especially refined sugar, so it's important to find a healthy alternative. Agave is extracted from the Agave plant.

Lucuma from a Peruvian fruit, it contains iron, vitamin B3 beta-carotene and phosphorus, has a very low sugar content and has a light biscuit flavor.

Xylitol is extracted from the bark of the birch tree and has 40% of the calories of sugar and is not cariogenic.

Stevia from the plant by the same name, it has a strong sweetening power 10/15 times that of sugar, and does not contain any sugar. The only problem is that it has a licorice aftertaste, so it may not appeal to everyone. Cost: from 6 to 12 euros for 250 gr.

Vitamin B12

The problem with the vegan diet is that we can run into a deficiency of vitamin B12 since it is found only in products of animal origin.

This can lead to various problems, including memory loss, elevated homocysteine which can lead to heart attacks, and problems with the nervous and motor systems, as well as depression and fatigue. The solution is to take vitamin B12 in tablets, but not just any tablet.

The solution is to take vitamin B12 in tablets, but not just any tablet.

In order for vitamin B12 to be absorbed it must be taken through sublingual tablets, that is, ones that dissolve under the tongue, because vitamin B12 alone is not absorbed through digestion.

Additionally there are two or three types of vitamin B12 tablets, cyanocobalamin, methylcobalamin, and hydroxocobalamin.

Although the latter appears to be the closest to B12 found in food, the easiest to find and best to take as an oral supplement is methylcobalamin. This is because cyanocobalamin does not offer, from studies done, the advantages that it should be able to offer, and is not absorbed in an optimal way. Additionally, as the name suggests, cyanocobalamin has a cyanide molecule, which the body must eliminate. It appears that the suggested dose of methylcobalamin is 1000mcg and up. Here is a link to further explore this topic.

http://www.dadamo.com/B2blogs/blogs/index.php/2004/02/07/cyano

cobalamin-versus-methylcobalamin?blog=27

I can suggest you google for methylcobalamine sublingual

Tips for saving and basic preparations for recipes.

There are some basic preparations and tips that will help you indulge your imagination and create recipes by combining sauces that you will find in this book and spend less.

The first preparation is the zucchini pasta, Buy some green zucchini (if they are not organic I recommend removing the green peel with a potato peeler) and pass them in the spiralizer and your pasta is done, no cooking, no electricity costs or gas! Consider a large and a half or two courgettes per person.

You can do the same thing with carrots, cleaning them well with a knife or peeler before using the spiralizer.

Another fundamental preparation is raw couscous or rice. Take some cauliflower (organic in this case if you can) clean it well, cut it and put it in the blender. Turn the blender on and off until it reaches a consistency similar to couscous or rice. You can also add lemon juice to enhance the flavor and freshness.

Bananas are a great foundation for any smoothie. You can add some spinach or other vegetables with a bland flavor and get a great smoothie full of vitamins and minerals. A great smoothie is made with 2 bananas, a handful of blueberries and a handful of spinach.

Add water to taste.

Never centrifuge bananas, you get too little juice.

Search the internet for a fruit and vegetable wholesaler in your city that also sells at retail and buy us the necessary for the whole week, you will spend even less than at the supermarket, even spending only 6/7 euros a day to eat.

Do you fancy ice cream? Put some fresh fruit cut into pieces in the freezer (ripe bananas are great for this). Blend them alone or with homemade almond or hazelnut milk, Another great way to save and improve your raw food is to do sprouting.

Coconut oil and cocoa butter are used in many recipes

Recipes!

Here are a few recipes to get you started. Recipes are intended per person

Guacamole

1 ripe avocado

½ large onion or one small onion

1 tomato

1/2 or 1 lime (as preferred)

2 cloves of garlic

a pinch of cumin
coriander seeds

salt

Clean the avocado and mash the pulp until it becomes a puree.

Finely chop the onion, garlic and tomato and add them to the avocado. Squeeze the lime and add the juice as well. Add the cumin, coriander and salt.

Excellent on its own or as a sauce for zucchini or carrot pasta. In this case you can add a drop of water to stretch the sauce.

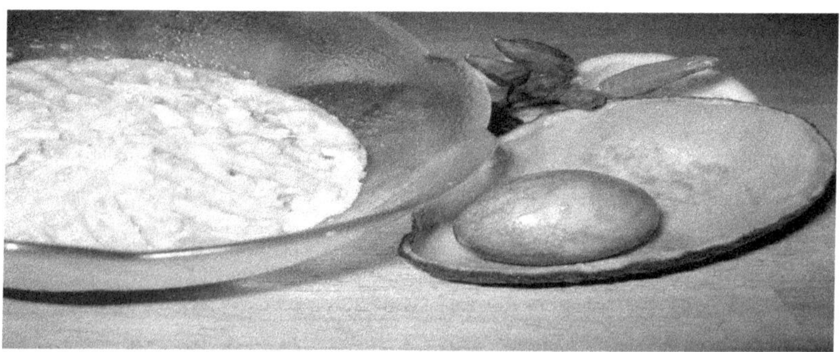

Raw cheese

1 cup of walnuts or sunflower seeds or cashews soaked overnight ½ cup of water

½ teaspoon of salt

1 tablespoon of lemon

fresh or dried herbs to cover the cheese Blend the nuts or seeds adding water if necessary until you reach a creamy and smooth consistency.

Squeeze out the excess water with a piece of linen clean Create cheese molds and roll them in herbs

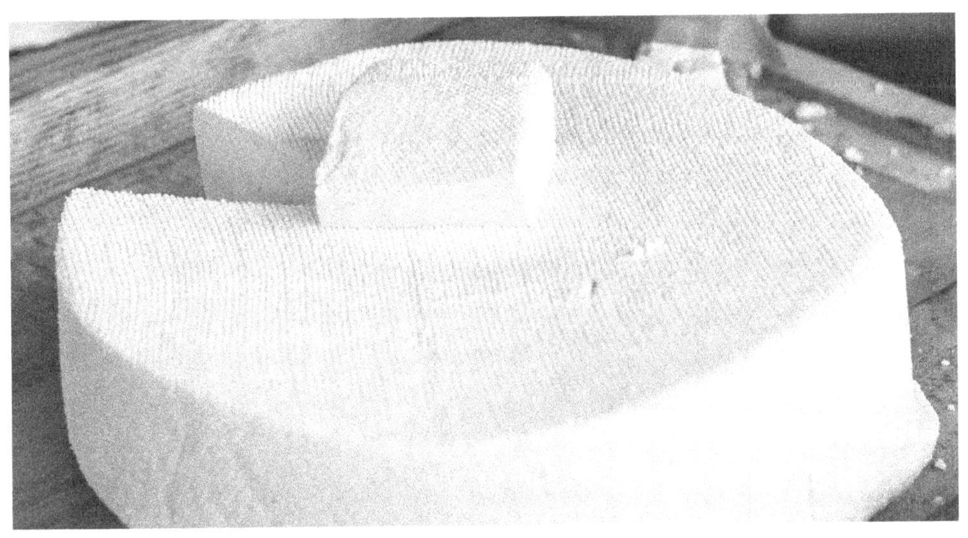

Salad dressing

1/3 cup of olive oil

lemon juice and zest (only the yellow part) 3 tablespoons of agave
juice

1 tablespoon of soy sauce

2 tablespoons of black olives
3 cloves of garlic blend everything

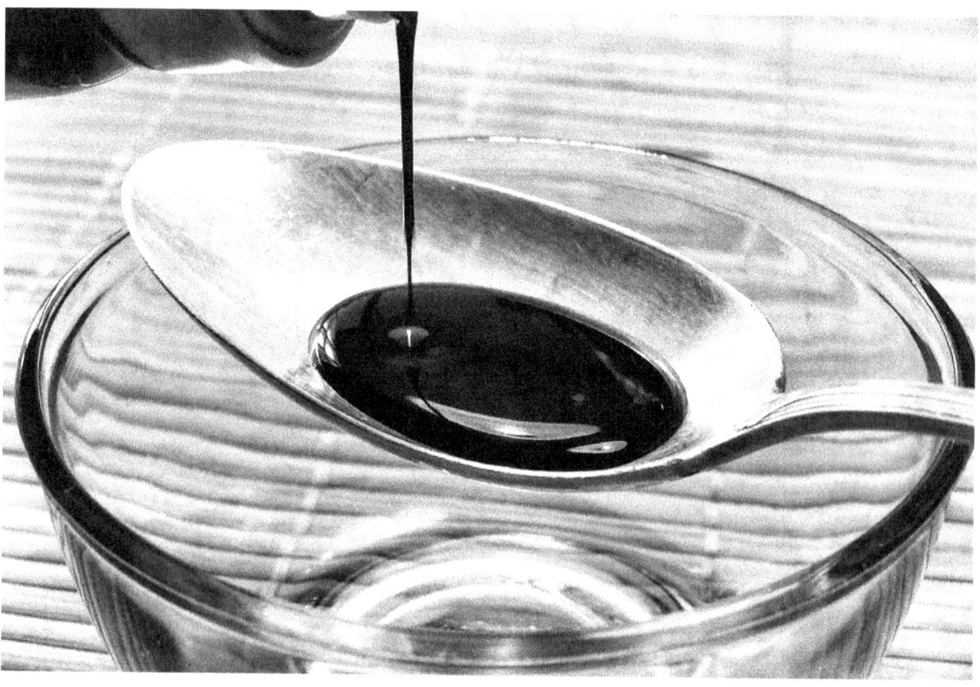

Broccoli with cheese 1 cup broccoli, tips without stems 20 gr sunflower seeds

3 tablespoons nutritional yeast

3 tablespoons of extra virgin olive oil (optional: rosemary)

a spoonful of tahini

the juice of 1 lemon

a spoonful of tamari

salt

Wash the broccoli and separate the buds and put them in a bowl. Mix the salt, tamari, 2 tablespoons of oil and lemon juice in a bowl and pour over the broccoli.

Massage for a couple of minutes and leave to rest for at least 10

minutes.

Meanwhile, put the sunflower seeds, the nutritional yeast, a tablespoon of oil and the rosemary in the blender and blend well.

The basic raw cheese will be obtained in this way. Optionally it can be modified by adding other spices such as chili for example.

Drain the excess liquid from the broccoli and add the cheese and mix.

Add the tahini to the broccoli with a little water and nutritional yeast to taste

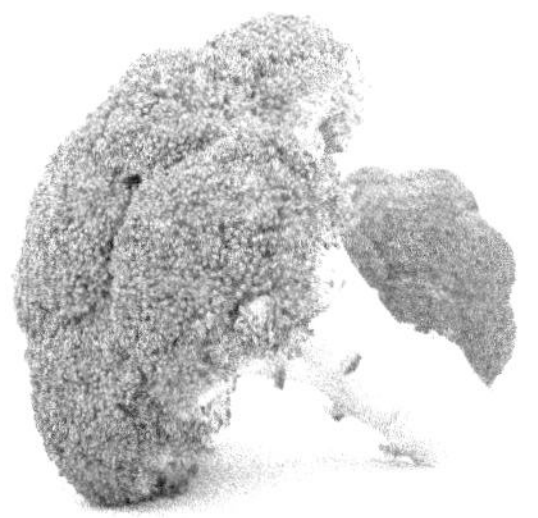

Spaghetti with tomato sauce

2 zucchini

2 tomatoes

1 dried tomato

2 tablespoons of extra virgin olive oil 1 tablespoon of lemon

1 date

1 clove of garlic

salt

pepper

basil and / or chilli pepper to taste Create the zucchini pasta with the spiralizer. For the sauce, blend the fresh tomatoes, dried tomatoes, oil, lemon, date and garlic clove together with the chilli and / or basil.

Pour over the pasta and add salt and pepper and mix.

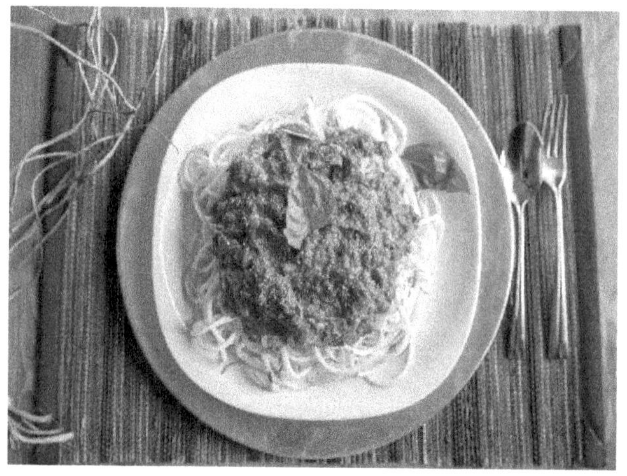

Spaghetti with pesto sauce

1 or 2 courgettes

a bunch of basil

50 gr of pine nuts or sunflower seeds 3 tablespoons of extra virgin olive oil 1 tablespoon of flaky nutritional yeast salt

Wash and clean the courgettes and possibly peel them, if they are not organic. Pass them in the spiralizer to create the spaghetti.

Blend well the pine nuts (or sunflower seeds for a cheaper recipe) with the oil, basil, nutritional yeast and a pinch of salt.

Pour the sauce over the zucchini pasta and mix well.

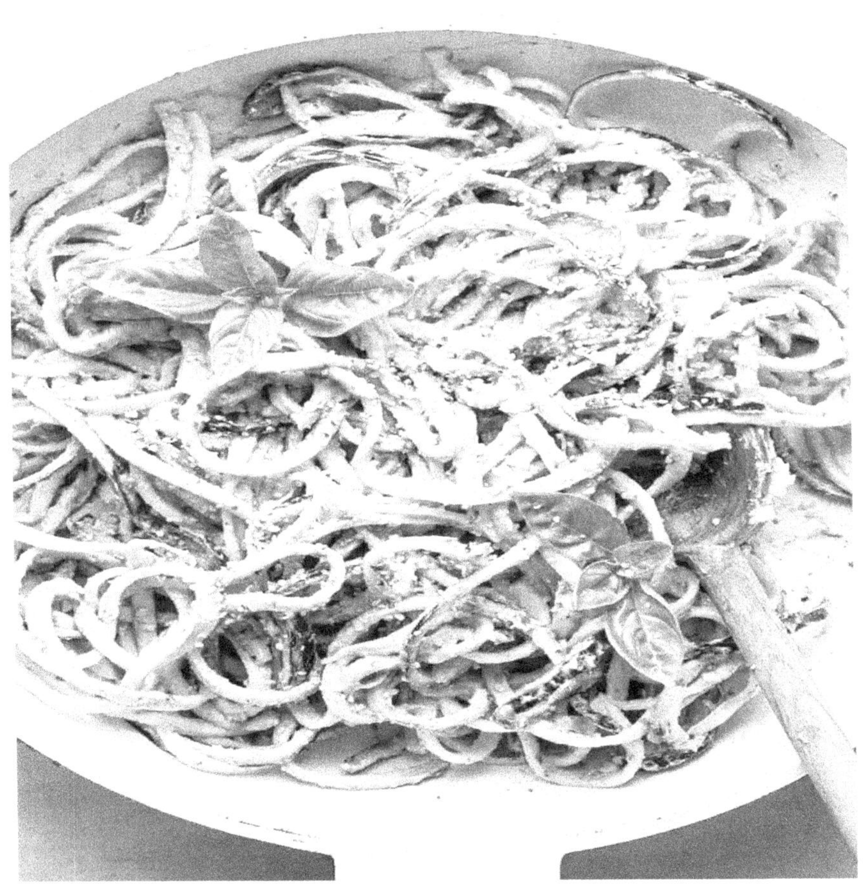

Raw Caponata

1 eggplant

coarse salt

2 tomatoes

4 chopped dried tomatoes (previously soaked for at least half an hour in cold water)

1 ½ tablespoons of raisins

1 tablespoon of chopped celery

½ tablespoon of capers (not necessarily raw food) 2 tablespoons of extra virgin olive oil 2 tablespoons of agave juice

2 tablespoons of lucuma powder

2 tablespoons of crumbled walnuts or pine nuts ½ tablespoon of lemon juice

1 tablespoon of soy sauce or nama shoyu 1 tablespoon of chopped green olives a handful of chopped basil leaves black pepper

Peel and cut the eggplant into cubes and put it under the coarse salt for an hour.

Put the rest of the ingredients on a plate and mix. (wash capers and olives are often too salty) Add the eggplant after having drained it, washed and squeezed it to remove excess salt

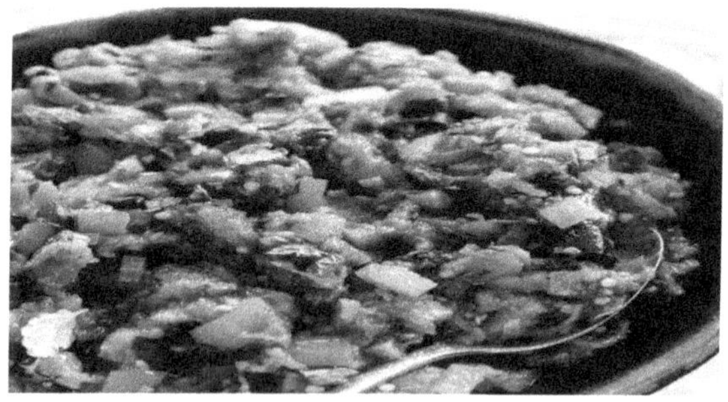

Raw Peperonata

1 red pepper

½ yellow pepper

½ orange or green pepper

4 dried tomatoes (previously soaked for at least half an hour in cold water)

1 tomato

1 sprig of basil

¼ onion

1 clove of garlic

1 pinch of oregano

4 tablespoons of extra virgin olive oil salt

chilli and cayenne pepper to taste Cut the washed and seeded peppers into strips and add the oil and salt. Massage them briefly and leave them for 10 minutes to macerate. Meanwhile, blend the tomato with the dried tomatoes and the garlic clove. Add everything to the peppers. Also add the finely chopped onion, basil and oregano. Drain the excess liquid and add the chilli and cayenne pepper if necessary.

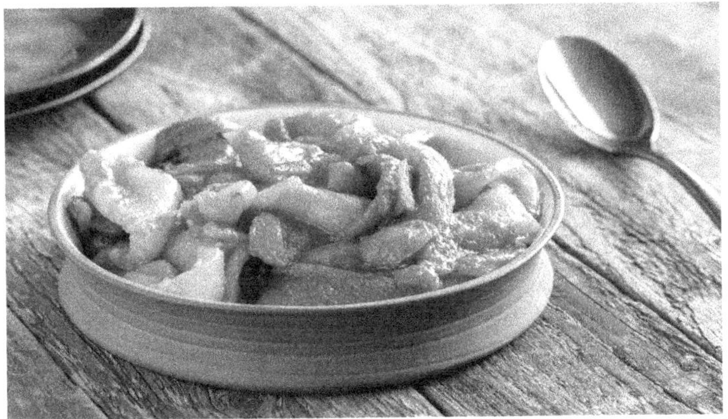

Raw Pad Thai

2 carrots

1 or 2 zucchini

1 tablespoon of tahini

1 tablespoon of tamari

1 tablespoon of extra virgin olive oil 1 small, ripe avocado

1 teaspoon of chopped red pepper

½ tablespoon of agave juice

 a handful of hazelnuts

Pass the carrots and zucchini in the spiralizer after washing them.

Blend or mix in a bowl the tahini, tamari, oil, agave juice and half of the chilli.

Mix the sauce with the pasta and add the avocado cut into small pieces.

Sprinkle the paste with chopped hazelnuts and a pinch of red pepper

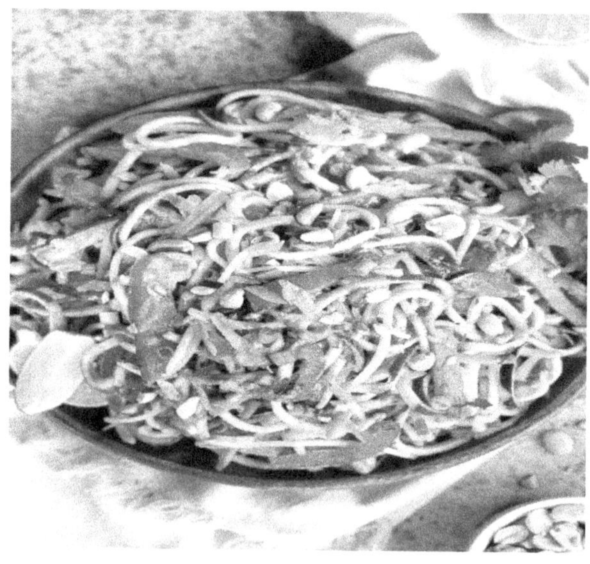

Spaghetti or Rice with Curry For the sauce:

1 avocado

½ teaspoon of lime juice

½ teaspoon of lemon juice

1 tablespoon of coriander seeds or fresh coriander ½ tablespoon of curry

½ cm of ginger root

little pepper or chili

2 tablespoons of water

For the Pasta: 1 1/2 courgettes

or

For the Rice: half a cauliflower

Blend all the sauce ingredients. Separately blend the cauliflower for the rice or pass the zucchini in the spiralizer and pour the sauce and mix

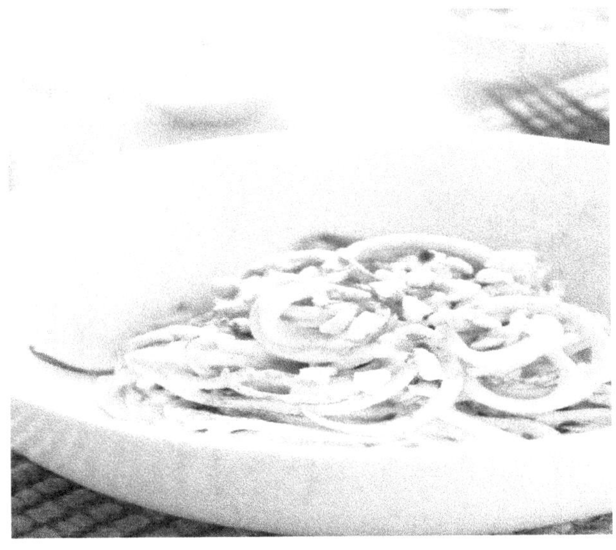

Raw Hamburgers This recipe would ideally need a dryer, but I tried it without a dryer and I must say that it is still good!

½ cup of fresh and dried mushrooms left to soak for a while 1 tablespoon of extra virgin olive oil 1 pinch of cumin

1 tablespoon of tamari

1 cup total of sunflower seeds, walnuts and almonds 1 cup in total of parsley, red onion and red pepper 1 clove of garlic

1 pinch of fresh rosemary

1 pinch of chopped red pepper

salt and pepper

Blend the sunflower seeds, walnuts and almonds first. Add the rest of the ingredients little by little and blend well. Shape the dough with your hands to form burgers. Put in the dryer for 3 or 4 hours or eat without drying, with seasoned rocket as a side dish

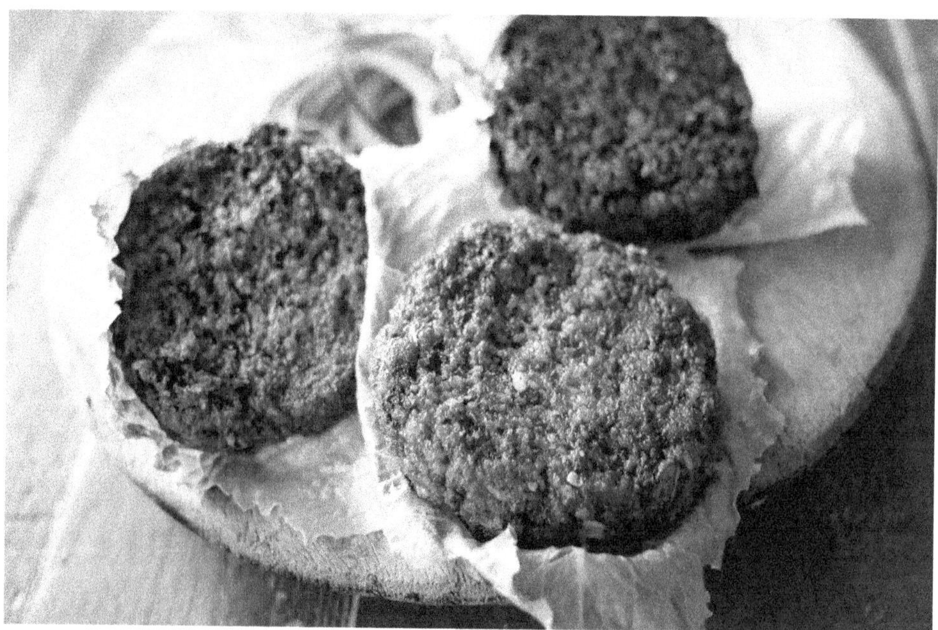

Apple pie

3 dates

a handful of sunflower seeds, almonds or walnuts ½ tablespoon of carob powder

1 green apple

cinnamon

1 teaspoon of agave juice (non-raw) or similar Blend or chop the seeds or almonds or nuts finely. (you can also blend them less fine if you prefer a little consistency in the base of the cake). Add the dates without the stone and the carob powder and blend. It will turn out a dough that you can flatten on a plate with your hands to form thebase of the cake. Blend or cut the apple into small pieces (without making it a puré) adding the agave juice and cinnamon to taste and spread it all on the base of the cake. You can eat it like this or have it cool in the upper shelf of the fridge for an hour or two.

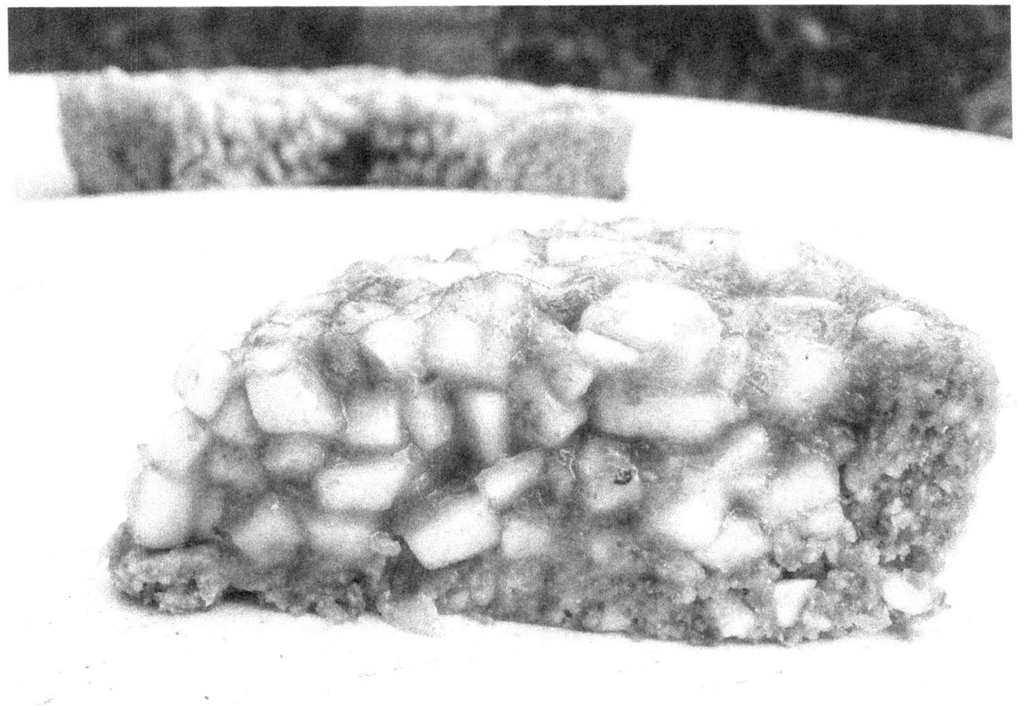

Chocolate Bon Bons

½ cup of almonds

½ cup of dates (previously soaked in water for an hour) 2 tablespoons of carob powder (or raw cocoa powder) 1 or 2 teaspoons of agave juice

to taste two cardamom seeds or a little chilli (optional: a tablespoon of coconut oil)

blend or put the almonds in the coffee grinder. Add the dates, carob and agave juice. If you like, add the cardamom or chilli. Blend everything until you get a sticky dough and shape it into balls with your hands. Especially you put the coconut oil and leave it in the fridge for an hour. .

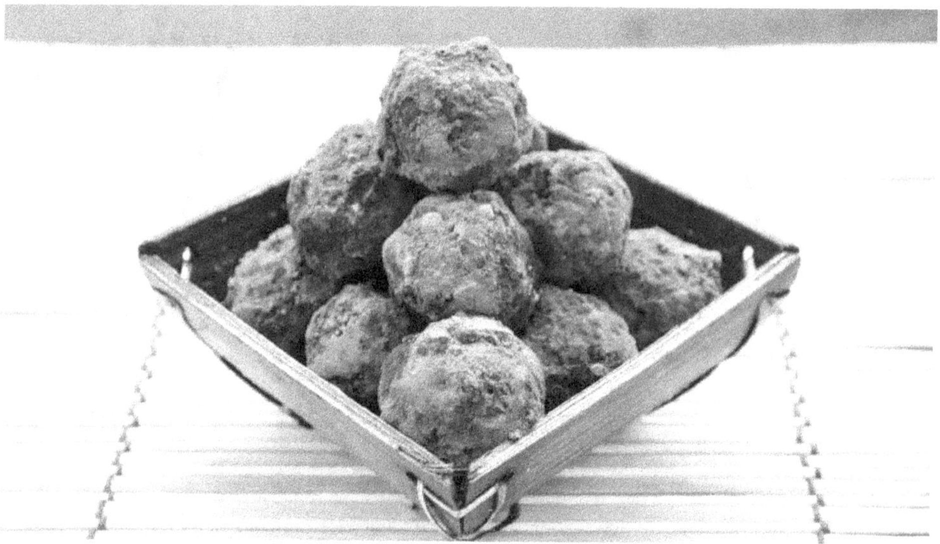